Weight Watchers Freestyle Cookbook

The Newly Weight Watchers Zero Point Freestyle Cookbook with Smart Point Recipes for Rapid Weight Loss and Keeping Healthy

By Malee Harlon

CONTENT

Introduction

The Weight Watchers Freestyle Plan changes every year by bringing out new reforms in different categories. The Weight Watchers Freestyle plan brings out changes to itself which are going to be explained in the coming portions. The coming portions are going to clear out all your doubts regarding what has been removed, what has been added and of course all about the Weight Watchers Freestyle Zero Point Foods. The Weight Watchers Freestyle has been added with above 200 food items which don't need any tracking, weighing or measurement.

The major changes are being done to Zero Point Foods. This makes the Weight Watchers Freestyle not that hard to understand at all. One more major change is in the Roll Over Points, which can be changed from one day to the other without worrying at all. A lot of specs of the previous Weight Watchers Plan are still included in the Weight Watchers Freestyle 2019. These include the SmartPoints in which you can earn various points for different activities. Planning these SmartPoints makes your plan not only simpler and easy to follow, but also gives you the opportunity to make healthier choices in your diet plan.

Chapter 1 Weight Watchers Zero Point Freestyle Plan 2021

WW Zero Point Freestyle Overview

The new additions to The WW Zero Point Freestyle plan are given out as follows:

1. Apart from the already mentioned WW Zero Point Food changes, there are certainly other changes which are drafted to make the plan easier for you to hit your weight loss targets. You can use your unused daily Roll Over Points (max. 4 points) the next day for that every week.
2. As the week finishes up, if you haven't used these Roll Over Points, they are termed useless then and aren't rolled over for the upcoming week. This makes it easy to save these points along with your weekly points so that you can use them over at a particular day and maintain a healthy diet plan.
3. One major change is that the number of allowed Daily Points has reduced in this year's plan. This is because of the addition of various new Zero Point foods to the plan. The calculation approach for your daily points is still dependant on gender, age, weight, and height. You can grab this number either from the Weight Watchers website or from your Weight Watchers leader.
4. The technique of earning FitPoints has also changed on this year's plan. The previous technique for earning FitPoints wasn't even and people

would earn them at various rates. The reason for this is that many individuals would calculate them via scheduled exercise while others would prefer using an activity monitor. To make this uniform for everyone, FitPoints has offered 3,000 steps for ensuring everybody's fitness. This will make everybody start from the same point and earn their FitPoints at the same pace. Irrespective of whether you are using a pocket guide or a monitor, the calculation for FitPoints is the same.

5. The technique of swapping your FitPoints is also the same as the previous plans. It is solely up to you whether you want to swap them for some food or don't use it at all. There is no compulsion.

Similarities with the previous Weight Watchers Plans:

There are many things in The Zero Point Freestyle 2019 which are just like the previous WW plans. These include:

1. The SmartPoints are the basis of the Weight Watchers Plan. The plan is termed as a successful one due to the easy calculation and tracking of thee SmartPoints. The calculation technique for the SmartPoints is the same in this year's plan just like the previous ones. This means that the followers of the plan don't have to recalculate the nutritional values of the already included foods apart from the new additions. This also makes it easier for making recipes without any fear of calculations unless you are using the new Zero Point foods in them.

2. The goals for activity every week are also the same as the previous Weight Watchers plan. There is just as a light change in it in which everyone's fitness goals are starting with accomplishing 3,000 steps.

3. The tracking method for foods is also the same just like the previous plans. Keep in mind that you will still need to track, measure, calculate, and measure your food on the new plan too unless you are consuming the 'freebies'.

4. There is still a weekly and daily allowance for you to consume food items. It is up to you to swap your FitPoints for foods or not use them at all.

What are the SmartPoints and the Zero Points?

In the Weight Watchers plan, every food is allocated with a specific numerical value called **'SmartPoints'**. The SmartPoints are based on the basis of nutritional science and is used to measure the amount of food you consume. It makes you follow a healthy, nutritious, and smart diet plan to lose weight, have sound energy, and health. The SmartPoints are based on four factors i.e. protein, calories, sugar, and saturated fats. It works as follows:

- Proteins are responsible for lowering the SmartPoints Value
- Sugar and saturated fats increment the SmartPoints value.
- Calories are responsible for declaring the total worth of SmartPoints food has.

Zero Point Foods, on the other hand, don't have any SmartPoint value and can be utilized for a day or so. They are basically described as BFD on the WW Freestyle Plan.

What are the advantages of Zero Point Foods?

There are numerous benefits of Zero Point Foods. As there are many new additions to this list, the followers of the plan aren't going to be much worried about tracking, measuring, calculating the messed up points of these foods. You can have various blends with different foods allowed on the Zero Point Freestyle 2019 program and make your diet menu versatile. Simply combine any Zero Point Food with a food item having a certain SmartPoint and you can track it just by adding the SmartPoints and ignoring the Zero Point Food to have a blended recipe for yourself.

Prior to the introduction of Zero Point Foods to the Weight Watchers Freestyle plan, these food items were tested clinically for trial purposes and it yielded a lot of promising results for the diet planners. While these trials were being conducted, the following observations were made:

- The hunger and cravings of the participants of these tests were observed to be low and the cravings for food were becoming lower because of having less hunger.
- In a short time span of merely 5 months, approximately 3 out of every 4 participants declared the diet plan perfect for weight loss as they achieved their results.
- A huge 93% of the individuals involved in the tests declared the Freestyle plan to be more promising and successful and made them feel healthier than any other diet plan of similar type.
- 82% of those participants who had previously gone through various weight loss diet plans considered the Freestyle plan to be easier and convenient to adapt.
- A whopping 93% participant stated that this program gave them more food choices and independence than any other weight loss program and yet was able to achieve their desired results.

New Zero Point Foods

As we have previously stated that The Weight Watchers Freestyle has done some changes for this year. The purpose of these changes is to make you understand and used to with alterations and promote 'Freestyle'. Without these changes, you will be stuck with the same old plan, which is going to bore you out very soon. Before you proceed with The Newly

Weight Watchers Freestyle, you clearly need to have a look at the changes to the Zero Point Food category. These changes are explained as follows:

Zero Point Veggies:

If you are a Weight Watchers Freestyle follower, you must have known that most of the fruits and veggies were classified as the Zero Points foods. The Weight Watchers Freestyle Cookbook also classifies them similarly but with some additions. These include the following additions:

➤ Peas and Sweet corn are added to the Zero Point category so you don't have to worry about tracking, weighing or measuring them.
➤ There has been an addition of a few starchy veggies to the vegetable category for Zero Point foods which is very exciting for the diet plan followers. These include lentils and beans.
➤ Foods like pinto beans, black beans, chickpeas, and many more have been classified as Zero SmartPoints valued items.

It is important to understand that if you are getting these foods in a canned form, sternly make it sure that there is no added sugar or oil in it. In case of added oils and sugar, calculate the points according to the nutrition table given on the can. In case of any ambiguity or doubt, simply scan the nutrition label on the cam with you Weight Watchers mobile app to get more accurate results and see if they are Zero Point Foods or not.

Non-Zero Point Veggies:

Just like the addition of various veggies to Zero Point foods of The Newly Weight Watchers Freestyle plan, there are certain veggies which weren't included in the Zero Points category for this year. These include the following:

➤ All dried veggies are considered Non-Zero Point Foods as they are considered to be 'snacks' which can be over consumed easily.

➤ Potatoes are also categorized as Non-Zero Point Foods for similar reasons as mentioned above.

You need to carefully calculate your points while consuming them to follow the plan perfectly.

Zero Point Meats:

There hasn't been any meat on the Weight Watchers Plan previously as a Zero Point food. This is one of the major change in The Newly Weight Watchers Freestyle plan which is making people go crazy about it. The important thing to note down is that not every lean meat has made it to the Zero Point list for The Weight Watchers Freestyle plan; rather it only includes turkey and chicken. Keep in mind the following important tips for Zero Point meats:

➤ Both the chicken and turkey should be 'skinless' for categorizing it as Zero Point Foods for The Newly Weight Watchers Freestyle plan.

➤ Lean turkey breasts and chicken breasts thinly sliced deli meats also carry Zero Points on the points list. You can serve yourself with ground lean chicken and ground lean turkey as much as you want as they have also made it to the list of Zero Point Foods.

If these meats are used in a certain recipe, the Weight Watchers recipe calculator will automatically use the Zero Point values for these items. In case you are manually calculating the points, you have to strike off the nutrition value of turkey or chicken from the point calculation.

Non-Zero Point Meats:

Just like any food category, some lean meats weren't graded as Zero Point Foods. These include:

➤ Lean beef and pork are categorized as Non-Zero Point foods. The reason for their non-inclusion as Zero Point Foods is that a healthy and sound diet includes the limitation of red meat consumption in a week. As the weight Watchers program is based on promoting a healthy diet plan around the world, red meat has been credited with points which need to be calculated.

➤ Dried Meats like jerky are also categorized in this portion. The reason for their inclusion is that they are considered as 'snacks' which can be over-consumed. This is why you have to keep a track of how much you have to eat.

You need to carefully calculate your points while consuming them to follow the plan perfectly.

Zero Point Seafood and Fish:

➤ Despite the fact that some fish are having a high-fat content, all the fish and seafood is categorized as Zero Point foods for The Weight Watchers Freestyle 2019 plan. They are included because fish and seafood are high in nutrients and are a must for a healthy diet plan which is the basis of the Weight Watchers program.

It is important to understand that if you are getting these foods in a canned form, sternly make it sure that there is no added oil in it. Always prefer getting a canned fish with water in it instead of oil. In case of any ambiguity or doubt, simply scan the nutrition label on the cam with you Weight Watchers mobile app to get more accurate results and see if they are Zero Point Foods or not.

Non-Zero Point Seafood and Fish:

Despite the reason that all seafood and fish are classified as Zero Point foods, there are certain exceptions which need to be understood clearly. These include:

➢ All canned fish and seafood including oil in it are classified as Non-Zero Point foods.

➢ Just like dried meats, dried seafood and fish are also considered as Non-Zero Point foods. But, smoked fish is 'okayish' similarly like smoked turkey and smoked chicken breasts.

You need to carefully calculate your points while consuming them to follow the plan perfectly.

Zero Point Fruits:

The fruits category didn't get much change at all and almost similar to the previous Weight Watchers Freestyle programs. Just for mentioning:

➢ All the fruits, except a few, are classified as Zero Point Foods.

It is important to understand that if you are getting these foods in a canned form, sternly make it sure that there is no added sugar or oil in it. In case of added oils and sugar, calculate the points according to the nutrition table given on the can. In case of any ambiguity or doubt, simply scan the nutrition label on the cam with you Weight Watchers mobile app to get more accurate results and see if they are Zero Point Foods or not.

Non-Zero Point Fruits:

Although, all the fruits are considered as Zero Point foods, what didn't make the list for The Weight Watchers Freestyle 2019 plan is as follows:

➤ Just like the previous plans, plantains and avocados are still not the part of The Weight Watchers Freestyle plan for this year.

➤ Smoothies are also considered as a Non-Zero Point Food. Even if your smoothie is made with purely nothing but Zero Point foods, still you will need to calculate SmartPoints for it. It is because in the liquid form you might over consume the yogurt and fruits without having the feeling of being full.

You need to carefully calculate your points while consuming them to follow the plan perfectly.

Other New Zero Point Foods:

There are certain new additions to The Weight Watchers Freestyle 2019 plan's Zero Point foods. There are various reasons for the induction of these new Zero Point foods. The reasons range from the nutritional benefits these food offers, promote a healthy lifestyle and are tended to be eaten in a moderate quantity. These new Zero Point foods include the following:

➤ Eggs
➤ Quorn and Tofu (meat substitute)
➤ Both Greek and regular, non-fat yogurt (plain)

It is important to note that whenever you are grabbing a yogurt for yourself, make it sure that it falls under the restrictions put by The Weight Watchers Freestyle 2019 plan. Make sure to grab non-fat and unsweetened (plain) yogurt. In case the yogurt is sweetened or having a slight amount of fats, you are required to calculate the points to follow the plan perfectly.

Non-Zero Point Foods:

There are certain foods which didn't make it to the Zero Point food list for The Weight Watchers Freestyle 2019 plan. These include:

➢ Non-fat soft cheeses like the non-fat cottage cheese are classified as Non-Zero Point foods despite having similarities to yogurt. It is because not only they are over consumed by people but also carry a larger amount of calories than the latter.

Zero Point Food List

Apples	Corn (yellow, white, on the cob, kernels, baby ears)
Applesauce (unsweetened)	Daikon
Artichokes heart	Dates, fresh
Arrowroot	Egg whites
Artichokes	Egg substitutes
Asparagus	Egg whole, including yolks
Arugula	Edamame (shelled or pods)
Banana	Eggplant
Bamboo shoots	Escarole
Figs, fresh	Endive
Beans (all varieties)	Fennel
Beets	Fish (all varieties, including smoked)
Beans, canned, fat-free, refried	Fruit salad
Berries (all varieties) Broccoli rabe	Fruit cup, unsweetened
Broccoli	Fruit cocktail
Broccoli Slaw	Fruit, unsweetened
Brussels sprouts	Grapes
Broccolini	Ginger root
Cabbage (all varieties)	Melon balls
Cauliflower	Grapefruit
Cantaloupe	Garlic
Caviar	Guavas
Celery	Greens (all varieties)
Carrots	Guavas, strawberries
Cherries	Honeydew melon
Cucumber	Hearts of palm
Chard (all varieties)	Jerk chicken breast
Calamari	Jack fruit
Chicken breast (99% fat-free)	Jerusalem artichokes (sun chokes)
Collard	Jerk chicken breast
Clementines	Jicama
Cranberries	Kohlrabi
Chicken breast or tenderloin (boneless, skinless or with bone)	Kiwifruit
Coleslaw mix (packaged, shredded)	Kumquats

Lychees	Pumpkin
Lemon	Pomelo
Lettuce (all varieties)	Radishes
Lentils	Radicchio
Leeks	Rutabagas
Lemon zest	Raspberries
Lime zest	Salad, side without dressing
Lime	Salad, mixed greens
Mung Daal	Salad tossed without dressing
Mung bean sprouts	Salad, three beans, without sugar or oil
Mangoes	Salad, fat-free (all varieties)
Mushrooms (all varieties)	Scallions
Mushroom caps	Satay chicken without peanut sauce
Nori seaweed	Sashimi (all varieties)
Nectarines	Seaweed
Okra	Sauerkraut
Onions	Strawberries
Oranges (all varieties)	Star fruit
Passion fruit	Spinach
Parsley	Shellfish (all varieties)
Papayas	Shallots
Peaches	Squash (all varieties)
Pea Shoots	Sprouts (all varieties)
Pears	Tofu (all varieties including smoked)
Peas (all varieties)	Taro
Peas and carrots	Tangerines
Pepperoncini	Tangelo
Peppers (all varieties)	Tomatillos
Persimmons	Tomato (all varieties)
Pico de gallo	Tomato sauce
Pickles, unsweetened	Tomato puree
Pimientos, canned	Turkey breast (99% fat-free)
Plumcots	Turnips
Pineapples	Turkey breast or tenderloin (boneless, skinless or with bone)
Plums	Vegetable, stir-fried without sauce
Pomegranates	Vegetable, mixed
Pomegranate seeds	Watercress
Pumpkin puree, unsweetened	Water chestnuts
Watermelon	Yogurt, plain, fat-free, unsweetened (all varieties including soy and Greek)

All the veggies and fruits are fresh (cooked and raw), drained, or frozen, canned without oil or sugar. All the seafood and poultry are frozen, fresh (cooked or raw), canned in SmartPoints values spices sauces, without any added oil.

Tips for Zero Point Freestyle Plan

Although the Weight Watchers Freestyle Plan for this year isn't complicated at all and can be followed conveniently without any hurdle. Yet, we have drafted out various tips for you to follow the plan in an effective manner. These tips are as follows:

1. Stay Hydrated:

This tip is too easy to adapt and doesn't really need much effort. It takes some time to generate a regular intake of water. You can enhance your hydration levels by having a higher fruit intake. But, ultimately you have to keep your water levels up.

2. Keep your snacks in easily accessible locations:

Whenever your hunger strikes in, you always tend to grab anything worth eating to kill that hunger. For this, keep healthy snacks in easily accessible locations to eat them whenever you get hungry.

3. Boost your supply of Herbs:

Always have an ample supply of spices and herbs in your reach. You can grow them at your own house or even grab them in a container from a store. These herbs add a lot of flavor to your food and that too without the addition of any undesired calories.

4. Go for new experiences:

We will recommend experiencing new recipes and foods on the plan apart from the ones you are already used to. This is going to pave a way for new foods into your diet plan, making it more versatile.

5. Cut down high-calorie foods into smaller portions:

Cutting a high-calorie food into smaller portions will help you out in expending an excessive effort to get your hands on every piece as compared to getting a bigger, single portion. For instance, while consumption, small pieces of cheese will take more time and efforts than an entire big block of it. Your fill is going to be faster if you are having a thought about reaching far ahead.

6. Prefer wearing tight clothes:

Whenever we are eating, our bellies tend to expand. It is recommended to wear tight clothes while eating to make weight loss effective and possible. The idea is based on the fact that you are going to stop eating while your clothes get uncomfortable for you due to tightness.

7. Bring Doggie bags to home:

This is the most exciting tips of all. Instead of eating all your allowed food in a restaurant, bring some of it back to your home for later consumption. This is not only going to control your diet but also lets you have two meals at a single price. You can further make it easy for yourself by convincing your waiter for splitting it into two portions, one packed and one served.

8. Maintain your shelves properly and stocked:

It is a drastic thing to experience while being on any weight loss plan that you aren't having any healthy food item in your shelf. We recommend stacking up and prepping your meals beforehand for the coming week to avoid any mishap and urge to have takeout.

9. Don't resist your cravings:

You shouldn't be resisting your cravings, but have a moderate approach while doing so. When you resist a craving, you always consume a bunch of unnatural substitutes for it before ending u eating what you desired in the first place. Avoid doing this, maybe a small portion of chocolate isn't that much of a danger as much as your unnatural substitutes.

10. Plan your goals and have rewards for it:

It is very promising to set a certain goal and reward yourself upon achieving it to keep yourself motivated. Make these goals a bit harder whenever you feel like they are becoming too easy to achieve.

11. Food logging is important:

Logging down your eating habits is a very important thing to observe and maintain your diet plan. Log down properly whatever you eat and also the amount you eat. It will stop you from eating things that aren't allowed on the plan.

12. Have a check of your body:

Take photos of your body in the initial stages and then after some days compare your body to the previous pictures. Check for yourself how much have you succeeded and how much more you want to accomplish with your diet plan. This is going to keep you motivated.

13. Understand portion sizes:

It is important to understand the size of every serving and then remain stick to it. Don't slip out of the restrictions of portion sizes else your plan isn't going to work out properly. These portion sizes are going to make you understand your diet more effectively.

Chapter 2 Breakfast Recipes

Pineapple Juice

Prep Time: 10 Minutes, Cook Time: 0 Minutes

Servings: 6

Smart Points: 4 points

Ingredients

- 5 cups fresh pineapple, chopped
- 1½ cups water
- 2 pinches salt

Directions:

1. Mix together all the ingredients and pour in a high-speed blender.
2. Pulse until smooth and strain the juice in 6 serving glasses.

Nutritional Information per Serving:

Calories: 68; Fat: 0g; Protein: 0.7g; Sugar: 13.5g;

Dates Quinoa

Prep Time: 10 Minutes, Cook Time: 15 Minutes

Servings: 4

Smart Points: 5 points

Ingredients

- 1 cup red quinoa, dried
- ¼ teaspoon vanilla extract
- ¼ teaspoon ground cinnamon
- 2 dates, pitted and finely chopped
- 2 cups unsweetened almond milk
- ½ cup fresh strawberries, hulled and sliced

Directions:

1. Put almond milk, quinoa, vanilla and cinnamon in a pan over low heat.
2. Cook for about 13 minutes stirring occasionally.
3. Serve garnished with strawberries.

Nutritional Information per Serving:

Calories: 179; Fat: 0.2g; Protein: 5.7g; Sugar: 3.5g;

Green Veggie Smoothie

Prep Time: 10 Minutes, Cook Time: 0 Minutes

Servings: 2

Smart Points: 1 point

Ingredients

- ¼ cup fresh spinach
- ½ cup green cabbage, chopped
- 1½ cups chilled water
- ½ cup broccoli florets, chopped
- 1¼ drops liquid stevia, to taste
- ½ cup small green bell pepper, seeded and chopped

Directions:

1. Mix together all the ingredients and pour in a high-speed blender.
2. Pulse until smooth and pour the juice in 2 serving glasses.

Nutritional Information per Serving:

Calories: 20; Fat: 0g; Protein: 1.3g; Sugars: 3.5g;

Eggs and Tomato Scramble

Prep Time: 10 Minutes, Cook Time: 15 Minutes

Servings: 3

Smart Points: 4 points

Ingredients

- ¼ cup fresh basil, chopped
- 4 eggs
- 1 tablespoon olive oil
- ¼ teaspoon red pepper flakes, crushed
- Salt and black pepper, to taste
- ½ cup grape tomatoes, chopped

Directions:

1. Whisk together eggs, salt, red pepper flakes and black pepper in a large bowl.
2. Add basil and tomatoes and mix well.
3. Heat oil in a non-stick skillet over medium-high heat and slowly add egg mixture.
4. Cook for 5 minutes continuously stirring and dish out to serve.

Nutritional Information per Serving:

Calories: 130; Fat: 2.5g; Protein: 7.7g; Sugars: 1.3g;

Berry Oatmeal

Prep Time: 5 Minutes, Cook Time: 25 Minutes

Servings: 8

Smart Points: *4 points*

Ingredients

- 1 cup fresh blackberries
- 2 cups dry oats
- 1 cup fresh cranberries
- 1 cup pecans, chopped
- 8 cups water
- 2 bananas, peeled and mashed

Directions:

1. Put oats and water in a large pan and boil over medium-high heat.
2. Lower the heat and let it simmer for about 15 minutes, occasionally stirring.
3. Dish out in a serving bowl and keep aside to cool.
4. Stir in mashed banana and garnish with pecan and berries to serve.

Nutritional Information per Serving:

Calories: 131; *Fat:* 0.4g; *Protein:* 3.5g; *Sugars:* 5.3g;

Baked Cherry Pancakes

Prep Time: 15 Minutes, Cook Time: 22 Minutes,

Servings: 10

Smart Points: 6 points

Ingredients

- 1 cup unsweetened almond milk
- 2 teaspoons olive oil
- 6 eggs
- 2 pinches salt
- 1 cup whole-wheat flour
- 2 teaspoons vanilla extract
- ½ cup almonds, chopped
- ¼ teaspoon ground cinnamon
- 2 tablespoons butter, melted
- 4 cups fresh sweet cherries, pitted and halved

Directions:

1. Preheat the oven to 440 degrees F and grease an ovenproof skillet with olive oil.
2. Mix together cinnamon, whole-wheat flour and salt in a bowl.
3. Add almond milk, eggs, melted butter and vanilla extract and beat until well combined.
4. Combine flour mixture with egg mixture until well mixed.
5. Arrange cherries on the bottom of the ovenproof skillet in a single layer.
6. Sift the flour mixture evenly over cherries and top with almonds.

7. Transfer the skillet into oven and bake for about 20 minutes.

8. Dish out from the oven and allow it to cool for at least 5 minutes.

9. Cut into equal sized wedges to serve.

Nutritional Information per Serving:

Calories: 180; *Fat:* 2.7g; *Protein:* 5.8g; *Sugars:* 0.5g;

Yogurt & Granola Bowl

Prep Time: 15 Minutes, Cook Time: None

Servings: 8

Smart Points: 3 points

Ingredients

- 4 cups fat-free plain Greek yogurt, divided
- ½ cup fresh blueberries
- 1 cup fresh strawberries, hulled and sliced
- ½ cup crunchy maple granola
- ½ cup fresh raspberries

Directions:

1. Mix together blueberries, strawberries and raspberries in a bowl.
2. Divide 2 cups of yogurt evenly in 8 parfait glasses and top with berries.
3. Place remaining yogurt over berries evenly in each parfait.
4. Top with granola and immediately serve.

Nutritional Information per Serving:

Calories: 99; *Fat:* 0g; *Protein:* 12.6g; *Sugars:* 3.6g;

Eggs with Spinach

Prep Time: 15 Minutes, Cook Time: 25 Minutes

Servings: 4

Smart Points: 3 points

Ingredients

- ¼ cup scallion, chopped
- Salt and black pepper, to taste
- 2 tablespoons extra-virgin olive oil
- 10 cups fresh baby spinach, chopped
- 4 eggs

Directions:

1. Preheat the oven to 390 degrees F and grease a baking dish.
2. Put oil and scallion over medium high heat in a skillet.
3. Cook for about 5 minutes and add spinach, salt and black pepper.
4. Cook for 5 more minutes and transfer the spinach mixture into a baking dish.
5. Make 4 holes in the spinach mixture and crack 1 egg in each hole.
6. Bake for about 15 minutes and serve garnished with parsley.

Nutritional Information per Serving:

Calories: 97; *Fat:* 1.4g; *Protein:* 7.8g; *Sugars:* 1.2g;

Strawberry and Plum Smoothie

Prep Time: 10 Minutes, Cook Time: 0 Minutes

Servings: 4

Smart Points: 4 points

Ingredients

- 2 cups green tea, brewed and cooled
- ½ cup ice cubes, crushed
- 2 medium plums, pitted and chopped
- 4 cups frozen strawberries, hulled
- 1 cup unsweetened almond milk

Directions:

1. Put all the ingredients in an immersion blender and pulse until smooth.
2. Pour into 4 glasses and immediately serve.

Nutritional Information per Serving:

Calories: 75; *Fat:* 0g; *Protein:* 0.5g; *Sugars:* 4.5g;

Mushroom Omelette

Prep Time: 15 Minutes, Cook Time: 25 Minutes,

Servings: 6

Smart Points: 3 points

Ingredients

- ½ cup red bell peppers, seeded and chopped
- ½ cup onions, chopped
- Salt and black pepper, to taste
- ½ cup unsweetened almond milk
- 2 tablespoons chives, minced
- 8 large eggs
- ½ cup fresh mushrooms, sliced

Directions:

1. Preheat the oven to 360 degrees F and grease a pie dish lightly.
2. Whisk together eggs, almond milk, salt and black pepper until mixed well.
3. Mix together onions, bell peppers and mushrooms in another bowl.
4. Pour the egg mixture in the pie dish and top evenly with vegetable mixture.
5. Top with chives and transfer the pie dish in the oven.
6. Bake for about 25 minutes and remove from oven.
7. Top with remaining tomatoes and immediately serve.

Nutritional Information per Serving:

Calories: 107; Fat: 2.1g; Protein: 8.9g; Sugars: 1.5g

Sausage Quiche

Prep Time: 15 Minutes, Cook Time: 25 Minutes

Servings: 8

Smart Points: 7 points

Ingredients

- ½ cup Parmesan cheese, shredded
- 8-ounce turkey sausages
- 12 eggs, lightly beaten
- 2 cups zucchini, shredded
- ½ cup fat-free milk
- ½ cup low-fat mozzarella cheese, shredded
- 2 red bell peppers, seeded and chopped
- Salt and black pepper, to taste

Directions:

1. Preheat the oven to 330 degrees F and lightly grease a pie plate.
2. Put the sausages, zucchini and bell pepper in a skillet.
3. Cook for about 8 minutes and dish out the sausage mixture into a bowl.
4. Stir in the Parmesan cheese and spread the mixture evenly into prepared pie plate.
5. Whisk together eggs, milk, salt and black pepper in a bowl.
6. Pour egg mixture over the turkey sausage mixture.
7. Top with mozzarella cheese and transfer into the oven.
8. Bake for about 25 minutes and dish out to serve hot.

Nutritional Information per Serving:

Calories: 218; Fat: 4.9g; Protein: 16g; Sugars: 3.3g;

Ham Muffins

Prep Time: 15 Minutes, Cook Time: 20 Minutes

Servings: 2

Smart Points: 3 points

Ingredients

- 2 eggs
- 2-ounce cooked ham, crumbled
- ¼ cup red bell peppers, seeded and chopped
- ½ tablespoon water
- Salt and black pepper, to taste
- ¼ cup onions, chopped

Directions:

1. Preheat the oven to 365 degrees F and grease 2 cups of a muffin tin.
2. Whisk together eggs, water, salt and black pepper until mixed well.
3. Add onions, bell peppers and ham and pour the mixture equally in prepared muffin cups.
4. Transfer into the oven and bake for about 20 minutes.
5. Dish out to serve hot.

Nutritional Information per Serving:

Calories: 120; Fat: 2.2g; Protein: 10.6g; Sugars: 1.7g;

Vanilla Crepes

Prep Time: 15 Minutes, Cook Time: 8 Minutes

Servings: 4

Smart Points: 4 points

Ingredients

- 1 tablespoon olive oil
- 2 tablespoons arrowroot powder
- Salt, to taste
- 4 eggs
- 1 teaspoon vanilla extract
- 2 tablespoons almond flour
- ½ teaspoon ground cinnamon

Directions:

1. Mix arrowroot powder, almond flour, salt and cinnamon thoroughly in a bowl.
2. Beat together eggs and vanilla in another bowl.
3. Combine both the egg and flour mixtures and keep aside.
4. Heat oil in a non-stick pan and slowly add ¼ of the mixture.
5. Tilt the pan to coat the bottom evenly in a thin layer and cook for about 1 minute per side.
6. Repeat with the rest of the mixture and dish out to serve.

Nutritional Information per Serving:

Calories: 129; Fat: 2g; Protein: 6.1g; Sugars: 0.5g;

Apple Porridge

Prep Time: 10 Minutes, Cook Time: 5 Minutes

Servings: 4

Smart Points: 4 points

Ingredients

- 2 cups unsweetened almond milk
- ½ teaspoon vanilla extract
- 2 large apples, peeled, cored and grated
- 3 tablespoons sunflower seeds
- ¼ cup fresh blueberries

Directions:

1. Put milk, almond sunflower seeds, apples and vanilla extract over medium-low heat in a large pan.
2. Cook for about 5 minutes while occasionally stirring.
3. Dish out into serving bowls and garnish with banana slices.

Nutritional Information per Serving:

Calories: 123; Fat: 0.1g; Protein: 4.8g; Sugars: 9.1g;

Berry and Yogurt Bowl

Prep Time: 10 Minutes, Cook Time: 0 Minutes,

Servings: 6

Smart Points: 3 points

Ingredients

- 1 cup fresh raspberries
- 3 cups fat-free plain yogurt
- 1 cup fresh blueberries
- 2 teaspoons raw honey

Directions:

1. Combine together the honey and yogurt in a bowl.
2. Top with blueberries and raspberries and immediately serve.

Nutritional Information per Serving:

Calories: 100; Fat: 0g; Protein: 7.5g; Sugars: 5.7g;

Chapter 3 Main Course Recipes

Turkey and Beans Wrap

Prep Time: 20 Minutes, Cook Time: 15 Minutes,

Servings: 3

Smart Points: 3 points

Ingredients

- 1½ tablespoons tomato sauce
- 3 large butternut lettuce leaves
- 1/8 teaspoon garlic powder
- Salt and black pepper, to taste
- 3-ounce lean ground turkey
- 1/8 teaspoon ground cumin
- ¼ cup cooked black beans
- ¼ cup onions, minced
- 1½ teaspoons extra-virgin olive oil

Directions:

1. Put garlic powder, tomato sauce, onions, turkey, cumin, salt and black pepper in a bowl.
2. Heat oil in a large skillet over medium heat and add turkey marinade.

3. Cook for about 10 minutes and stir in beans.

4. Simmer for about 3 minutes on low heat and keep aside to cool.

5. Divide the turkey mixture evenly over the lettuce leaves and immediately serve.

Nutritional Information per Serving:

Calories: 121; Fat: 0.9g; Protein: 9.3g; Sugars:3.9g;

Chicken and Salsa Chili

Prep Time: 15 Minutes, Cook Time: 8 Hours

Servings: 7

Smart Points: 5 points

Ingredients

- 2 cups salsa
- 1 onion, chopped
- 1 pound boneless chicken breast
- 2 garlic cloves, minced
- 1½ cups water
- 1 jalapeño pepper, minced
- 1 teaspoon ground cumin
- 3 green bell peppers, seeded and chopped
- 1 avocado, peeled, pitted and chopped
- 2 teaspoon chili powder
- Salt and black pepper, to taste

Directions:

1. Mix together chicken, water, salsa, garlic, cumin, salt and black pepper in a slow cooker.
2. Cover the lid and cook on LOW for about 6 hours.
3. Put onions, bell peppers and jalapeño pepper in a non-stick skillet.
4. Cook for about 5 minutes until well roasted and dish out the chicken.
5. Shred it with forks and return the chicken to slow cooker.
6. Stir in chili powder, avocado, roasted vegetables, salt and black pepper.

7. Cover the lid and cook for about 2 hours on LOW.

8. Dish out in a bowl and serve hot.

Nutritional Information per Serving:

Calories: 176; Fat: 1.8g; Protein: 18g; Sugars: 5.5g;

Chicken with Cranberries

Prep Time: 20 Minutes, Cook Time: 20 Minutes,

Servings: 6

Smart Points: 4 points

Ingredients

- 2 tablespoons fresh ginger, minced
- 1½ pounds skinless, boneless chicken thighs
- 1 cup fresh cranberries
- 2 tablespoons olive oil, divided
- 1 cup chicken broth
- ¼ cup onion, chopped finely
- 2 tablespoons unsweetened applesauce
- Salt and black pepper, to taste

Directions:

1. Put oil, chicken, salt and black pepper over medium heat in a large skillet.
2. Cook for about 5 minutes per side and dish out the chicken into a large bowl.
3. Put the onions in the same skillet and sauté for about 3 minutes.
4. Add broth and cook for about 5 minutes until boiled.
5. Stir in the cranberries and cook for about 5 minutes.
6. Season with salt and black pepper and drizzle with applesauce.
7. Cook for about 2 minutes and top with cranberry mixture to serve.

Nutritional Information per Serving:

Calories: 185; Fat: 1.3g; Protein: 25.9g; Sugars: 0.4g;

Turkey and Veggie Casserole

Prep Time: 15 Minutes, Cook Time: 50 Minutes,

Servings: 8

Smart Points: 5 points

Ingredients

- 2 medium zucchinis, sliced
- 1 cup tomato sauce
- 2/3 pound lean ground turkey
- 2 medium tomatoes, sliced
- 1 large onion, chopped
- 2 egg yolks
- ½ cup low-fat cheddar cheese, shredded
- 1 tablespoon fresh rosemary, minced
- 2 garlic cloves, minced
- 2 cups low-fat cottage cheese, shredded
- Salt and black pepper, to taste

Directions:

1. Preheat the oven to 490 degrees F and grease a large pan.
2. Place tomato slices and zucchini into prepared pan and transfer into the oven.
3. Bake for about 12 minutes and dish out to keep aside.
4. Put turkey in a non-stick skillet and cook for about 5 minutes.
5. Stir in the tomato sauce and cook for about 3 minutes.
6. Reduce the temperature of oven to 360 degrees F.

7. Arrange the turkey mixture into a baking dish and top with roasted vegetables.

8. Mix together rest of the ingredients in a bowl and spread cheese mixture evenly over vegetables.

9. Bake for about 30 minutes and dish out to serve hot.

Nutritional Information per Serving:

Calories: 181; Fat: 2.4g; Protein: 19.4g; Sugars: 2.7g;

Stir-Fried Shrimps

Prep Time: 15 Minutes, Cook Time: 5 Minutes,

Servings: 4

Smart Points: 4 points

Ingredients

- 2 tablespoons tamari
- Salt and black pepper, to taste
- ½ pound raw jumbo shrimp, peeled and deveined
- 1 tablespoon extra-virgin olive oil
- 2 garlic cloves, minced

Directions:

1. Put oil and garlic in a large skillet over medium heat.
2. Sauté for about 1 minute and add shrimp, salt, tamari and black pepper.
3. Cook for about 4 minutes and dish out to serve hot.

Nutritional Information per Serving:

Calories: 210; Fat:3g; Protein: 27g; Sugars:1.3g;

Squid with Eggs

Prep Time: 15 Minutes, Cook Time: 10 Minutes,

Servings: 3

Smart Points: 5 points

Ingredients

- 1 pound squid, cleaned and cut into rings
- 1 teaspoon olive oil
- ¼ yellow onion, sliced
- Salt, to taste
- 1 egg, beaten
- ¼ teaspoon ground turmeric

Directions:

1. Put oil and onions in a skillet over medium-high heat.
2. Sauté for about 5 minutes and add squid rings, salt and turmeric.
3. Allow it to simmer on medium-low heat for about 5 minutes and add beaten egg.
4. Cook for about 3 minutes and dish out to serve hot.

Nutritional Information per Serving:

Calories: 178; Fat:5.1g; Protein: 15g; Sugars:3.8g;

Grilled Cod

Prep Time: 12 Minutes, Cook Time: 8 Minutes,

Servings: 4

Smart Points: 4 points

Ingredients

- ½ teaspoon red pepper flakes
- 4 (4-ounce) cod fillets
- 1 tablespoon olive oil
- ½ teaspoon dried dill
- Salt and black pepper, to taste
- 1 tablespoon fresh lime juice

Directions:

1. Put all the ingredients in a bowl except cod and mix well.
2. Dredge the cod in the mixture and keep aside for about 1 hour.
3. Preheat the grill to medium-high heat and grease the grill grate.
4. Grill the cod fillets for about 4 minutes per side and dish out to serve hot.

Nutritional Information per Serving:

Calories: 82; Fat: 0.2g; Protein: 0.9g; Sugars: 4.5g;

Chapter 4 Salad Recipes

Tomato and Olive Salad

Prep Time: 15 Minutes, Cook Time: 0 Minutes,

Servings: 5

Smart Points: 5 points

Ingredients

- 1/8 cup red wine vinegar
- 2 large cucumbers, chopped
- ½ (2¼-ounce) can green olives, pitted and chopped
- 3 small tomatoes, chopped
- ¼ red onion, thinly sliced
- 2-ounce feta cheese, crumbled
- 1 (2½-ounce) can black olives, pitted and halved

Directions:

1. Put all the ingredients except red wine vinegar in a serving bowl.
2. Sprinkle with red wine vinegar and immediately serve.

Nutritional Information per Serving:

Calories: 132; Fat: 2.6g; Protein: 3.5g; Sugars: 4.2g;

Cucumber and Egg Salad

Prep Time: 12 Minutes, Cook Time: 0 Minutes,

Servings: 2

Smart Points: 4 points

Ingredients

For Salad

- 1 medium cucumber, cut spirally
- 1 hard-boiled egg, peeled and chopped
- ¼ cup celery, chopped

For Dressing

- ½ garlic clove, minced
- Salt and black pepper, to taste
- 1/3 cup fat-free plain Greek yogurt
- ¼ tablespoon Dijon mustard

Directions:

1. Put all the dressing ingredients in a large bowl and beat well.
2. Mix together cucumber, eggs and celery in a large serving bowl.
3. Drizzle the dressing over salad and toss to mix well.
4. Serve immediately.

Nutritional Information per Serving:

Calories: 109; Fat: 1.3g; Protein: 3.4g; Sugars: 3.8g;

Kale Salad

Prep Time: 10 Minutes, Cook Time: 0 Minutes,

Servings: 4

Smart Points: 4 points

Ingredients

- 2 scallions, chopped
- 2 red onions, sliced
- 2 fresh tomatoes, sliced
- 2 tablespoons fresh lemon juice
- 8 cups fresh kale, trimmed and chopped
- 4 tablespoons fresh orange juice
- 2 tablespoon almonds, chopped

Directions:

1. Mix together all the ingredients except almonds in a large bowl and toss to coat well.
2. Cover and refrigerate to marinate for about 8 hours.
3. Take out from the refrigerator and top with almonds to serve.

Nutritional Information per Serving:

Calories: 127; Fat: 0.2g; Protein: 6.1g; Sugars: 5.7g;

Radish & Carrot Salad

Prep Time: 15 Minutes, Cook Time: 0 Minutes,

Servings: 8

Smart Points: 4 points

Ingredients

For Salad

- 2 cups radishes, trimmed, peeled and julienned
- 6 cups carrots, peeled and julienned
- 1 cup fresh parsley, chopped

For Dressing

- 4 teaspoons coconut aminos
- 2 teaspoons fresh ginger, finely grated
- Salt, to taste
- ½ teaspoon garlic, minced
- 2 tablespoons olive oil
- 4 tablespoons balsamic vinegar
- 4 teaspoons raw honey

Directions:

1. Put all the salad ingredients in a large bowl and combine thoroughly.
2. Mix together all the dressing ingredients in a small bowl and combine.
3. Drizzle the dressing over salad and toss to coat well.
4. Dish out in small bowls and serve immediately.

Nutritional Information per Serving:

Calories: 88; Fat: 0.5g; Protein: 1.2g; Sugars: 7.6g;

Chicken Salad

Prep Time: 20 Minutes, Cook Time: 0 Minutes,

Servings: 8

Smart Points: 7 points

Ingredients

For Dressing

- ¼ cup fresh lemon juice
- ½ teaspoon fresh ginger, minced
- 4 tablespoons olive oil
- Salt and black pepper, to taste
- 4 tablespoons Dijon mustard

For Salad

- 6 cups chicken, shredded
- 1 small pineapple, peeled, cored and thinly sliced
- 1 cup scallions, sliced thinly
- 8 plum tomatoes, sliced thinly lengthwise
- 3 pounds Napa cabbage, shredded

Directions:

1. Mix together all the dressing ingredients in a small bowl until well combined.
2. Put all the salad ingredients in a large serving bowl and top with the dressing mixture.
3. Toss to coat and immediately serve.

Nutritional Information per Serving:

Calories: 291; Fat: 2.1g; Protein: 35.2g; Sugars: 9.5g;

Bulgur & Veggie Salad

Prep Time: 20 Minutes, Cook Time: 5 Minutes,

Servings: 6

Smart Points: 7 points

Ingredients

- 1 cup boiling water
- 1 cup bulgur
- 1 cup frozen edamame, shelled
- ½ pound red cherry tomatoes, halved
- ½ pound yellow cherry tomatoes, halved
- 1 cup scallion, chopped
- 2 tablespoons fresh dill, chopped
- 1 cup fresh parsley, chopped
- 1/3 cup fresh mint leaves, chopped
- ¼ cup extra-virgin olive oil
- ¼ cup fresh lemon juice
- Salt and black pepper, to taste

Directions:

1. Mix together bulgur and boiling water in a large heatproof bowl.
2. Cover and keep aside for at least 1 hour.
3. Put edamame in a pan of boiling water and cook for about 3 minutes.
4. Mix together cooked bulgur, edamame and remaining ingredients in a large bowl.
5. Keep at room temperature for at least 1 hour and serve.

Nutritional Information per Serving:

Calories: 212; Fat: 1.5g; Protein: 7.3g; Sugars: 2.3g;

Apple, Beet & Carrot Salad

Prep Time: 15 Minutes, Cook Time: 0 Minutes,

Servings: 8

Smart Points: 4 points

Ingredients

For Salad

- 1¾ cups Braeburn apple, peeled, cored and grated
- 1¾ cups beetroot, peeled and grated
- 1¾ cups carrots, peeled and grated

For Dressing

- 1 tablespoon fresh gingerroot, grated finely
- 1 tablespoon raw honey
- 3 tablespoons fresh lime juice
- 2 tablespoons extra-virgin olive oil

Directions:

1. Mix together all the salad ingredients in a large serving bowl.
2. Beat together all the dressing ingredients until well combined.
3. Drizzle the dressing over salad and gently toss to coat well.
4. Refrigerate for about 30 minutes before serving.

Nutritional Information per Serving:

Calories: 92; Fat: 1.3g; Protein: 1g; Sugars: 4.7g;

Turkey Salad

Prep Time: 20 Minutes, Cook Time: 0 Minutes,

Servings: 3

Smart Points: 4 points

Ingredients

For Salad:

- ½ zucchini, julienned
- 1 cup cooked turkey, cubed
- ½ carrot, peeled and shredded
- 2 radishes, trimmed and thinly sliced
- ½ small head iceberg lettuce, torn
- ½ small onion, chopped

For Dressing:

- 1 tablespoon fresh lemon juice
- 1½ tablespoons extra-virgin olive oil
- ½ teaspoon fresh ginger, minced
- ½ garlic clove, minced
- ½ teaspoon unsweetened applesauce
- 1½ tablespoons extra-virgin olive oil
- ½ teaspoon fresh ginger, minced
- ½ garlic clove, minced
- ½ teaspoon unsweetened applesauce
- ½ teaspoon Dijon mustard

Directions:

1. Mix together all the salad ingredients in a large bowl and keep aside.
2. Put all the dressing ingredients in a small bowl and beat until well combined.
3. Pour the dressing over the salad and stir well to combine.
4. Serve in small bowls.

Nutritional Information per Serving:

Calories: 162; Fat: 3.2g; Protein: 14.6g; Sugars: 1.2g;

Fruit and Spinach Salad

Prep Time: 15 Minutes, Cook Time: 0 Minutes,

Servings: 7

Smart Points: 6 points

Ingredients

- 1 mango, peeled, pitted and cubed
- 1 pound fresh pineapple, peeled and cut into chunks
- 2 papayas, peeled, seeded and cubed
- ¼ cup fresh mint leaves, chopped
- 10 cups fresh baby spinach
- 3 tablespoons fresh lime juice

Directions:

1. Put all the ingredients in a large serving bowl except spinach.
2. Cover and refrigerate to chill before serving.
3. Divide spinach in the serving plates and top evenly with salad to serve.

Nutritional Information per Serving:

Calories: 115; Fat: 0.2g; Protein: 2.6g; Sugars: 20.5g;

Marinated Tomato Salad

Prep Time: 15 Minutes, Cook Time: 0 Minutes,

Servings: 2

Smart Points: 6 points

Ingredients

For Marinade

- 1/8 cup olive oil
- Salt and black pepper, to taste
- 1 garlic clove, finely minced
- ½ tablespoon prepared pesto
- 1½ tablespoons balsamic vinegar

For Salad

- 1 cup red grape tomatoes, halved
- 1 cup yellow grape tomatoes, halved
- ¼ red onion, thinly sliced
- ½ head iceberg lettuce, torn
- 1½ tablespoons fresh parsley, minced

Directions:

1. Mix together all the marinade ingredients in a large serving bowl until well combined.
2. Add onions, tomatoes and parsley and mix completely with marinade.
3. Cover and refrigerate for about 4 hours.
4. Put tomato mixture on the lettuce in a large serving bowl.
5. Drizzle with the marinade and immediately serve.

Nutritional Information per Serving:

Calories: 175; Fat: 3.5g; Protein: 2.5g; Sugars: 3.4g;

Lettuce and Beet Salad

Prep Time: 15 Minutes, Cook Time: 0 Minutes,

Servings: 6

Smart Points: 5 points

Ingredients

- 2 tablespoons balsamic vinegar
- 10 cups fresh lettuce
- 4 beetroots, chopped
- Salt, to taste
- 4 tablespoons olive oil

Directions:

1. Mix together all the ingredients in a large serving bowl.
2. Toss to mix well and immediately serve.

Nutritional Information per Serving:

Calories: 123; Fat: 1.4g; Protein: 1.5g; Sugars: 6.3g;

Corn and Tomato Salad

Prep Time: 15 Minutes, Cook Time: 0 Minutes,

Servings: 4

Smart Points: 5 points

Ingredients

- 1/8 cup extra virgin olive oil
- 3 tablespoons shallots, minced
- 2 cups corn kernels
- Salt and black pepper, to taste
- 3 cups fresh cherry tomatoes, halved

Directions:

1. Mix together oil, vinegar, salt and black pepper in a bowl to make dressing.
2. Add tomatoes and corn and toss to coat well.
3. Serve immediately.

Nutritional Information per Serving:

Calories: 150; Fat: 1.1g; Protein: 3.9g; Sugars: 6.1g;

Pears and Greens Salad

Prep Time: 10 Minutes, Cook Time: 0 Minutes,

Servings: 6

Smart Points: 7 points

Ingredients

- 4 tablespoons apple cider vinegar
- Salt and black pepper, to taste
- 8 cups mixed fresh greens
- 2 large green apples, cored and sliced
- 2 tablespoons unsalted cashews

Directions:

1. Mix together cashews, apple, greens, salt and black pepper in a large serving bowl.
2. Drizzle with apple cider vinegar and immediately serve.

Nutritional Information per Serving:

Calories: 179; Fat: 1.6g; Protein: 3.3g; Sugars: 14.6g;

Arugula Salad

Prep Time: 13 Minutes, Cook Time: 0 Minutes,

Servings: 4

Smart Points: 2 points

Ingredients

- 1 teaspoon garlic clove, minced
- Salt and black pepper, to taste
- 3 cups fresh arugula
- ¼ cup fresh basil, chopped
- 1 tablespoon olive oil
- 1 tablespoon balsamic vinegar
- 2 medium ripe tomatoes, cut into slices

Directions:

1. Put garlic, olive oil, basil, vinegar, salt and black pepper in a small blender and pulse until smooth.
2. Mix together the remaining ingredients in a large serving bowl.
3. Drizzle with the dressing and mix to coat well.
4. Serve immediately.

Nutritional Information per Serving:

Calories: 47; Fat: 0.5g; Protein: 1g; Sugars: 2g;

Chapter 5 Snacks Recipes

Roasted Almonds

Prep Time: 10 Minutes, Cook Time: 15 Minutes,

Servings: 3

Smart Points: 3 points

Ingredients

- ¼ tablespoon water
- ½ cup almonds
- 1/8 teaspoon red chili powder
- Salt, to taste
- ¾ tablespoon unsweetened applesauce
- 1/8 teaspoon ground cinnamon
- 1/8 teaspoon cayenne pepper
- ¼ teaspoon olive oil
- 1/8 teaspoon ground cumin

Directions:

1. Preheat the oven to 360 degrees F and grease a baking sheet.
2. Arrange the almonds onto a baking sheet and transfer into the oven.
3. Roast for about 10 minutes and remove from the oven.

4. Microwave applesauce over high for about 45 seconds in a microwave safe bowl.

5. Remove from microwave and add water and oil.

6. Mix together all the spices in a bowl and remove the almonds from oven.

7. Mix almonds with the applesauce mixture and stir to combine well.

8. Arrange the almond mixture onto baking sheet in a single layer and season evenly with spice mixture.

9. Roast for about 4 minutes and dish out from the oven.

10. Keep aside to cool and serve.

Nutritional Information per Serving:

Calories: 102; Fat:1.3g; Protein:3.4g; Sugars:2.1g;

Spinach Chips

Prep Time: 20 Minutes, Cook Time: 10 Minutes,

Servings: 2

Smart Points: 1 point

Ingredients

- 1/8 teaspoon ground cumin
- Salt, to taste
- 1/8 teaspoon olive oil
- 4 cups fresh spinach leaves
- ¼ teaspoon paprika

Directions:

1. Preheat the oven to 340 degrees F and line a baking sheet with a parchment paper.
2. Mix together olive oil and spinach leaves in a large bowl.
3. Sprinkle with salt and spices and arrange the leaves onto prepared baking sheet.
4. Transfer the baking dish in the oven and bake for about 10 minutes.
5. Dish out and serve immediately.

Nutritional Information per Serving:

Calories: 18, Fat:0.1g, Protein:1.8g, Sugars:0.3g;

Cod Sticks

Prep Time: 20 Minutes, Cook Time: 15 Minutes,

Servings: 4

Smart Points: 3 points

Ingredients

- ¼ teaspoon cayenne pepper
- ½ cup almond flour
- ½ cod fillet, thinly sliced
- 1 egg
- Salt and black pepper, to taste
- 1 teaspoon dried parsley, crushed

Directions:

1. Preheat the oven to 360 degrees F and grease lightly a large baking sheet.
2. Whisk together eggs in a bowl and keep aside.
3. Mix together parsley, cayenne pepper, flour and salt in a bowl.
4. Dip the cod sticks in egg and then coat with dry flour mixture.
5. Arrange the cod sticks into prepared baking sheet and transfer into the oven.
6. Bake for about 12 minutes, flipping once in the middle way and serve immediately.

Nutritional Information per Serving:

Calories: 112; Fat:0.8g; Protein:6.9g; Sugars: 0.1g;

Parsnip Fries

Prep Time: 20 Minutes, Cook Time: 40 Minutes,

Servings: 8

Smart Points: 6 points

Ingredients

- 2½ pounds small parsnips, peeled and quartered
- 4 tablespoons olive oil
- 3 tablespoons fresh ginger, minced
- Salt and black pepper, to taste
- 1 teaspoon red chili powder

Directions:

1. Preheat the oven to 330 degrees F and grease a 13x9-inch baking dish lightly with olive oil.
2. Add rest of the ingredients and toss to coat well.
3. Cover the baking dish with a piece of foil and bake for about 40 minutes.
4. Remove from the oven and serve immediately.

Nutritional Information per Serving:

Calories: 174; Fat: 1.1g; Protein: 1.9g; Sugars: 6.9g;

Seeds Crackers

Prep Time: 15 Minutes, Cook Time: 12 Hours,

Servings: 3

Smart Points: 4 points

Ingredients

- ½ cup sunflower seeds
- ½ teaspoon unsweetened applesauce
- 1 cup water
- ½ cup flaxseeds
- ½ tablespoon fresh ginger, chopped
- 1/8 cup fresh lemon juice
- Salt, to taste
- ½ teaspoon ground turmeric

Directions:

1. Set a dehydrator at 115 degrees F and line a dehydrator tray with unbleached parchment paper.
2. Put sunflower seeds, flaxseeds and water in a bowl and soak overnight.
3. Drain the seeds and keep aside.
4. Put the drained seeds and remaining ingredients in a food processor.
5. Pulse until well combined and place the mixture onto prepared dehydrator tray.
6. Score the size of crackers with a knife and dehydrate for about 12 hours.
7. Dish out to serve immediately.

Nutritional Information per Serving:

Calories: 151; Fat: 1.3g; Protein: 5.3g; Sugars: 0.8g;

Quinoa Croquettes

Prep Time: 20 Minutes, Cook Time: 20 Minutes,

Servings: 6

Smart Points: 4 points

Ingredients

- ¼ cup frozen peas, thawed
- 1 large boiled potato, peeled and mashed
- 1/8 cup plus ½ tablespoon olive oil, divided
- 1 garlic clove, minced
- ½ cup cooked quinoa
- 1/8 cup fresh cilantro, chopped
- ¼ teaspoon paprika
- Salt and black pepper, to taste
- 1 teaspoon ground cumin
- 1/8 teaspoon ground turmeric

Directions:

1. Heat half of oil in a frying pan over medium heat and add garlic and peas.

2. Sauté for about 1 minute and transfer the peas mixture into a large bowl.

3. Add remaining ingredients and mix until well combined.

4. Make equal sized patties from the mixture and keep aside.

5. Heat remaining oil in a large skillet over medium-high heat and add croquettes in batches.

6. Fry for about 4 minutes on each side and dish out to serve warm.

Nutritional Information per Serving:

Calories: 120, Fat: 0.7g, Protein: 3.1g, Sugars: 0.7g,

Cheddar Biscuits

Prep Time: 20 Minutes, Cook Time: 15 Minutes,

Servings: 4

Smart Points: 6 points

Ingredients

- 2 pinches ginger powder
- 2 pinches garlic powder
- ½ cup low-fat sharp cheddar cheese, shredded
- 1/8 teaspoon baking powder
- 1/8 cup butter, melted and cooled
- 1/6 cup coconut flour, sifted
- 2 eggs

Directions:

1. Preheat the oven to 400 degrees F and line a large cookie sheet with foil paper.
2. Mix together coconut flour, garlic powder, baking powder and salt in a large bowl.
3. Whisk together eggs and butter in another bowl and keep aside.
4. Combine flour mixture with the egg mixture until well combined.
5. Stir in cheddar cheese and place the mixture onto prepared cookie sheets.
6. Transfer into the oven and bake for about 15 minutes until top becomes golden brown.
7. Serve warm.

Nutritional Information per Serving:

Calories: 142; Fat:7.2g; Protein:6.4g; Sugars: 0.2g;

Stir-Fried Shrimps

Prep Time: 13 Minutes, Cook Time: 7 Minutes,

Servings: 2

Smart Points: 3 points

Ingredients

- 2 tablespoons tamari
- ½ pound raw jumbo shrimp, peeled and deveined
- 1 tablespoon extra-virgin olive oil
- Salt and black pepper, to taste
- 2 garlic cloves, minced

Directions:

1. Put olive oil and garlic in a large skillet over medium heat.
2. Sauté for about 1 minute and add shrimp, tamari, salt and black pepper.
3. Cook for about 6 minutes and dish out to serve hot.

Nutritional Information per Serving:

Calories: 156, Fat:1g, Protein: 22.3g, Sugars:2.4g,

Spicy Popcorn

Prep Time: 15 Minutes, Cook Time: 5 Minutes,

Servings: 6

Smart Points: 6 points

Ingredients

- ½ teaspoon garlic powder
- 1 cup popping corn
- 6 tablespoons olive oil, divided
- Salt, to taste
- 2 teaspoons ground turmeric

Directions:

1. Put half of olive oil over medium-high heat in a pan and add popping corn.
2. Cover the pan tightly and cook for about 2 minutes, shaking the pan until corn kernels begin to pop.
3. Remove from heat and transfer into a large serving bowl.
4. Stir in the remaining olive oil and spices to serve.

Nutritional Information per Serving:

Calories: 183; Fat:2.1g; Protein:1.8g; Sugars: 0.1g;

Green Devilled Eggs

Prep Time: 15 Minutes, Cook Time: 20 Minutes,

Servings: 3

Smart Points: 4 points

Ingredients

- ½ medium avocado, peeled, pitted and chopped
- 1/8 teaspoon cayenne pepper
- 3 large eggs
- 1 teaspoon fresh lime juice
- 1/8 teaspoon salt

Directions:

1. Put eggs in a pan of water and cook for about 15 minutes.
2. Drain the water and allow them to cool completely.
3. Peel the eggs and slice them in half vertically.
4. Scoop out the yolks and transfer half of them into a bowl.
5. Stir in avocado, lime juice and salt in the bowl of yolks.
6. Mash with a fork until well combined and fill the egg halves with avocado mixture.
7. Sprinkle with cayenne pepper and serve immediately.

Nutritional Information per Serving:

Calories: 140, Fat: 2.9g, Protein: 7g, Sugars: 0.8g,

Chapter 6 Desserts Recipes

Chickpea Fudge

Prep Time: 20 Minutes, Cook Time: 1 Hour,

Servings: 3

Smart Points: 5 points

Ingredients

- 1/8 cup almond butter
- 1/8 cup unsweetened almond milk
- ¼ teaspoon vanilla extract
- ½ cup cooked chickpeas
- 2 dates, pitted and chopped
- ½ tablespoon cacao powder

Directions:

1. Preheat the oven to 360 degrees F and line a baking dish with parchment paper.
2. Put all the ingredients in a food processor except cacao powder.
3. Pulse until well combined and dish out the mixture into a large bowl.
4. Stir in cacao powder and pour the mixture into the baking dish.
5. Smooth the top surface and transfer the baking dish in the oven.

6. Bake for about 1 hour ad dish out.

7. Refrigerate for about 2 hours before serving.

Nutritional Information per Serving:

Calories: 146; Fat:0.4g; Protein:6.9g; Sugars: 7.1g;

Strawberry Soufflé

Prep Time: 20 Minutes, Cook Time: 12 Minutes,

Servings: 12

Smart Points: 2 points

Ingredients

- 1/8 cup fresh lemon juice
- 10 egg whites, divided
- 2/3 cup unsweetened applesauce, divided
- 36-ounce fresh strawberries, hulled

Directions:

1. Preheat the oven to 350 degrees F and grease 12 ramekins.
2. Pulse the strawberries in a blender until a puree forms.
3. Strain the puree into a bowl and discard the seeds.
4. Beat together 4 egg whites, lemon juice and 6 tablespoons of applesauce in a bowl.
5. Add rest of the applesauce while gradually beating and fold the egg whites gently into the strawberry mixture.
6. Pour the mixture evenly into the ramekins and arrange the ramekins in a baking sheet.
7. Transfer into the oven and bake for about 12 minutes.
8. Dish out to serve.

Nutritional Information per Serving:

Calories: 48; Fat:0g; Protein:3.6g; Sugars: 5.8g;

Blueberry Pudding

Prep Time: 20 Minutes, Cook Time: 0 Minutes,

Servings: 3

Smart Points: 6 points

Ingredients

- 1 teaspoon lime zest, freshly grated
- 1 small avocado, peeled, pitted and chopped
- 5 tablespoons water
- 1 cup frozen blueberries
- 10 drops liquid stevia
- ¼ teaspoon fresh ginger, freshly grated
- 2 tablespoons fresh lime juice

Directions:

1. Put all the ingredients in a blender except blueberries and pulse until smooth.
2. Pour into small serving bowls and refrigerate to chill before serving.

Nutritional Information per Serving:

Calories: 173; Fat:2.8g; Protein:1.8g; Sugars: 5.7g;

Glazed Banana

Prep Time: 15 Minutes, Cook Time: 5 Minutes,

Servings: 4

Smart Points: 5 points

Ingredients

- 2 tablespoons unsweetened applesauce
- 2 bananas, under-ripened, peeled and sliced
- 2 tablespoons olive oil
- ¼ teaspoon ground cinnamon
- 2 tablespoons water

Directions:

1. Beat together applesauce and water in a small bowl.
2. Put olive oil and banana slices in a pan and fry for about 2 minutes on each side.
3. Arrange the banana slices in a serving plate and drizzle applesauce mixture evenly over banana slices.
4. Keep aside to cool and sprinkle with cinnamon to serve.

Nutritional Information per Serving:

Calories: 116; Fat: 1.1g; Protein: 0.7g; Sugars: 8g;

Raspberry Ice-Cream

Prep Time: 20 Minutes, Cook Time: 0 Minutes,

Servings: 3

Smart Points: 4 points

Ingredients

- 1 cup fresh raspberries
- 2 tablespoons coconut, shredded
- ¼ small banana, peeled and sliced
- ¼ cup coconut cream

Directions:

1. Put all the ingredients in an immersion blender and pulse until smooth.
2. Pour the mixture into an ice-cream maker and process according to manufacturer's directions.
3. Transfer into an airtight container and freeze for at least 5 hours.
4. Stir after every 30 minutes and serve chilled.

Nutritional Information per Serving:

Calories: 87; Fat: 5.2g; Protein:1.2g; Sugars: 3.7g;

Prep Time: 10 Minutes, Cook Time: 0 Minutes,

Servings: 3

Smart Points: 7 points

Ingredients

- 1 tablespoon fresh lime juice
- ½ cup frozen pineapple chunks, thawed
- 7-ounce unsweetened almond milk
- Pinch of salt
- 2 cups frozen banana slices, thawed

Directions:

1. Line a glass baking dish with a plastic wrap.
2. Put all the ingredients in an immersion blender and pulse until smooth.
3. Transfer the mixture evenly into prepared baking dish.
4. Freeze for about 1 hour before serving.

Nutritional Information per Serving:

Calories: 138; Fat: 0.2g; Protein: 1.6g; Sugars: 21.1g;

Chocolaty Tofu Mousse

Prep Time: 20 Minutes, Cook Time: 0 Minutes,

Servings: 2

Smart Points: 3 points

Ingredients

- 1 teaspoon cocoa powder
- 1 teaspoon almonds
- ¾ banana, peeled and sliced
- 6-ounces firm tofu, drained

Directions:

1. Put all the ingredients in a food processor and pulse until smooth.
2. Pour into serving glasses and refrigerate for about 4 hours before serving.

Nutritional Information per Serving:

Calories: 107; Fat:0.9g; Protein:7.8g; Sugars: 6g;

Banana Custard

Prep Time: 20 Minutes, Cook Time: 25 Minutes,

Servings: 4

Smart Points: 2 points

Ingredients

- ¼ teaspoon vanilla extract
- 2 eggs
- 1 ripe banana, peeled and finely mashed
- 7-ounce unsweetened almond milk

Directions:

1. Preheat the oven to 360 degrees F and grease lightly 4 custard glasses.
2. Arrange the glasses in a large baking dish.
3. Mix together all the ingredients in a large bowl until well combined.
4. Divide the banana mixture in custard glasses and pour water in the baking dish.
5. Transfer into the oven and bake for about 25 minutes.
6. Remove the baking dish from the oven and serve the custard.

Nutritional Information per Serving:

Calories: 66; Fat:0.8g; Protein:3.3g; Sugars: 3.8g;

Blackberry Crumble

Prep Time: 20 Minutes, Cook Time: 45 Minutes,

Servings: 4

Smart Points: 5 points

Ingredients

- ¼ cup banana, peeled and mashed
- ¼ cup arrowroot flour
- ¼ cup coconut flour
- 3 tablespoons water
- 1½ cups fresh blackberries
- ¾ teaspoon baking soda
- ½ tablespoon fresh lemon juice
- 2 tablespoons butter, melted

Directions:

1. Preheat the oven to 320 degrees F and grease lightly a baking dish.
2. Put all the ingredients in a large bowl except blackberries and mix well.
3. Place blackberries at the bottom of the baking dish and sprinkle with flour mixture.
4. Transfer into the oven and bake for about 45 minutes to serve.

Nutritional Information per Serving:

Calories: 118; Fat:4.2g; Protein:2.3g; Sugars: 3.8g;

Yogurt Cheesecake

Prep Time: 20 Minutes, Cook Time: 35 Minutes,

Servings: 10

Smart Points: 4 points

Ingredients

- 6 drops liquid stevia
- ½ cup raw cacao powder
- 1 teaspoon vanilla extract
- 3 cups low-fat Greek yogurt
- 4 egg whites
- ¼ cup arrowroot starch
- 1/8 teaspoon salt

Directions:

1. Preheat the oven to 350 degrees F and grease lightly a 9-inch cake pan.
2. Put all the ingredients in a large bowl and mix well.
3. Pour the mixture evenly into prepared pan and transfer into the oven.
4. Bake for about 35 minutes and dish out.
5. Refrigerate to chill for about 3 hours and cut into equal sized slices to serve.

Nutritional Information per Serving:

Calories: 98; Fat:0.6g; Protein:4.6g; Sugars: 13.8g;

Conclusion

The Weight Watchers Freestyle Plan changes every year by bringing out new reforms in different categories. There are various changes in The Weight Watchers Freestyle 2019 and has been added with above 200 food items which don't need any tracking, weighing or measurement. The major changes are being done to Zero Point Foods. This makes the Weight Watchers Freestyle 2019 not that hard to understand at all. One more major change is in the Roll Over Points, which can be changed from one day to the other without worrying at all about the so-called messy calculations.

A lot of specs of the previous Weight Watchers Plans are still included in the Weight Watchers Freestyle 2019. These include the SmartPoints in which you can earn various points for different activities. The plan is not at all hard to follow and provides you with the best possible diet plan towards a healthy lifestyle. The Weight Watchers Freestyle has done some changes for this year. The purpose of these changes is to make you understand and used to with alterations and promote 'Freestyle'. Without these changes, you will be stuck with the same old plan, which is going to bore you out very soon.

CPSIA information can be obtained
at www.ICGtesting.com
Printed in the USA
LVHW101337220221
679652LV00008B/511